HEALTHY LIVING HACKS

Quick Tips For A Better Life

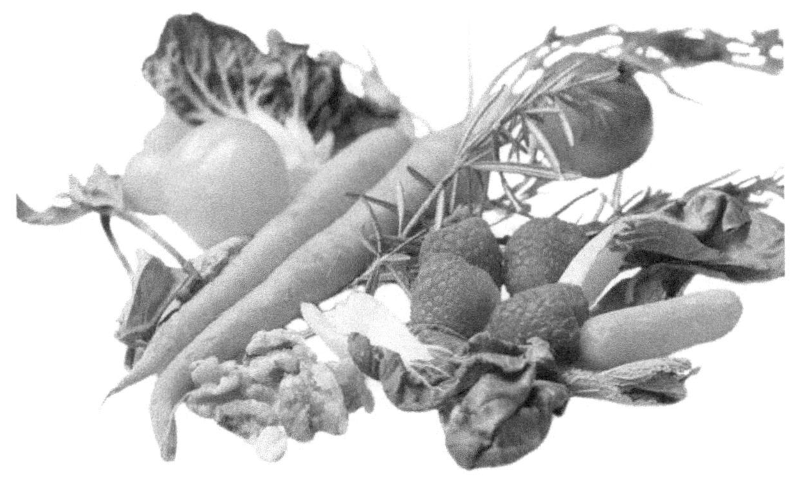

Susan Ribble

TABLE OF CONTENTS

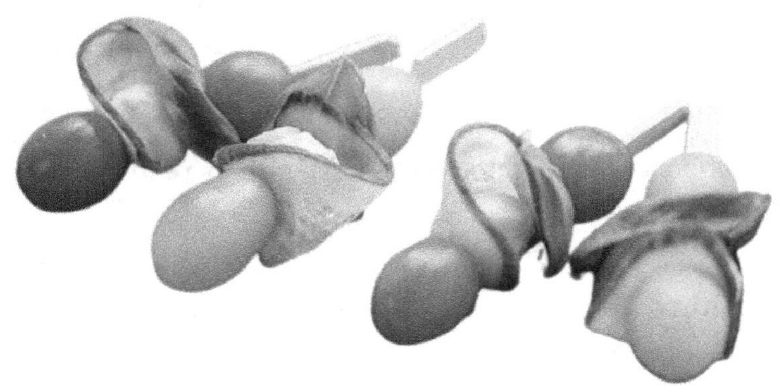

INTRODUCTION

Imagine waking up one morning to find yourself in a world where health is as effortless as breathing. No confusing diets, no overwhelming fitness regimes, just simple, effective tips that seamlessly fit into your daily routine. This world isn't a distant dream; it's within your reach, right here in the pages of this book.

"Healthy Living Hacks: Quick Tips for a Better Life" is your home. Think of this book as your personal guide on an exciting journey towards a healthier, happier you. We're not here to bombard you with scientific jargon or unrealistic expectations. Instead, we're offering a treasure trove of practical, quick tips that will transform your everyday habits into powerful health boosters.

Imagine you're at the crossroads of a bustling marketplace, filled with vibrant stalls offering the freshest produce, tantalizing aromas of home-cooked meals, and the invigorating buzz of people sharing their secret wellness hacks. You're handed a map, not just any map, but one that leads you to hidden gems – the best snack recipes, quick fitness routines, and mindful practices. Each stall you visit offers something new and delightful, making the journey as enjoyable as the destination.

As you stroll through this marketplace, you'll meet people just like you – busy professionals, parents juggling multiple roles, students striving for balance. They all have one thing in common: the desire to live a better, healthier life without sacrificing time or joy. These are the voices and stories that fill this book, offering real-life solutions to real-life challenges.

You will discover that healthy living does not necessitate drastic changes or a willpower that rivals your own. It's about making smart, small decisions that have a big effect. From quick breakfast hacks that kickstart your day with energy, to easy snacks that keep you going, and mindful moments that center your mind, each tip in this book is intended to fit easily into your life.

So, grab a cozy seat, perhaps a cup of your favorite herbal tea, and let's embark on this journey together. Flip through the pages, try out the tips, and watch as these simple hacks transform your life, one quick tip at a time. Welcome to the new, healthier, happier you!

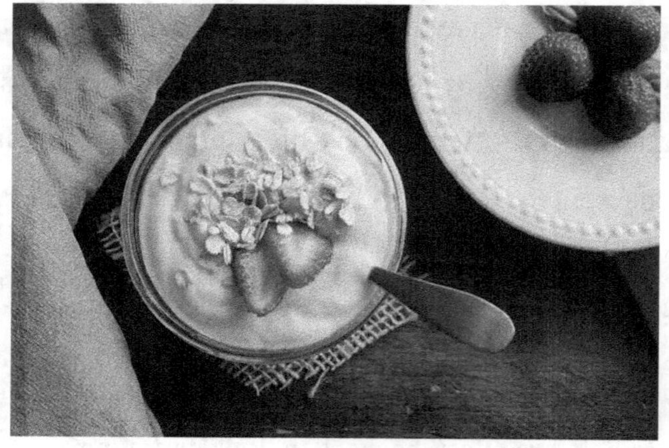

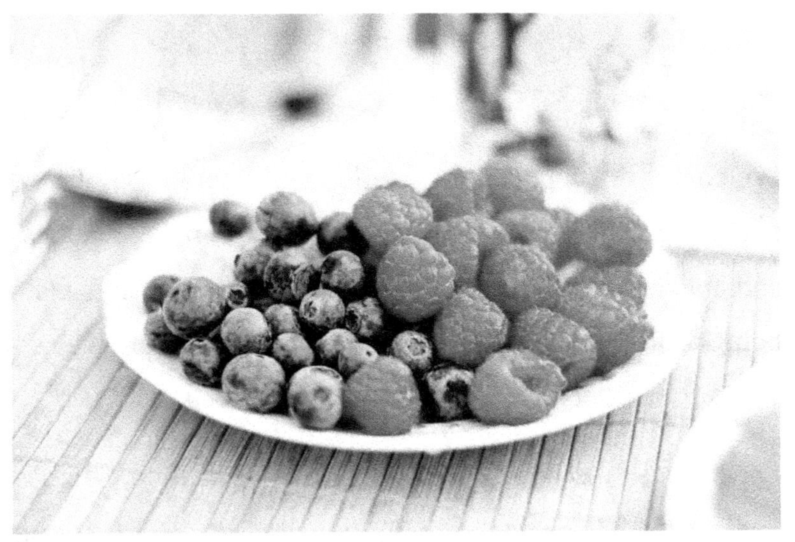

CHAPTER ONE

Superfoods for Everyday Health

Understanding Superfoods

Welcome to the vibrant world of superfoods! These nutritional powerhouses are packed with vitamins, minerals, and antioxidants that can supercharge your health and well-being. But what exactly are superfoods, and why are they so vital for our diets?

Superfoods are a unique classification of food sources tracked down in nature. By definition, they are calorie sparse and nutrient dense, meaning they pack a lot of punch in terms of nutrients but relatively few calories. They are superior sources of essential nutrients and antioxidants, which we require but cannot produce ourselves.

Think of superfoods as nature's ultimate gift to our health. From the vibrant blueberries bursting with antioxidants to the nutrient-dense kale leaves, superfoods provide us with the essential nutrients our bodies crave to function optimally. They help combat chronic diseases, improve brain function, and boost energy levels.

Incorporating Superfoods into Your Diet

Superfoods don't have to be difficult or time-consuming to include in your daily diet. Making little, reliable changes can prompt huge upgrades in your general wellbeing. Start your morning with a superfood smoothie by blending spinach, kale, or avocado with a handful of berries, a banana, and some almond milk. This quick and easy breakfast is packed with vitamins and minerals to kickstart your day.

Replace your usual snacks with superfood alternatives. Swap out potato chips for a handful of almonds or a piece of dark chocolate, both of which are rich in antioxidants and healthy fats. Add a handful of quinoa to your salads, mix chia seeds into your yogurt, or sprinkle flaxseeds over your oatmeal. These small additions can significantly boost the nutritional value of your meals.

Get creative with vegetables by incorporating a variety of colorful veggies into your diet. Try roasting sweet potatoes, making a stir-fry with broccoli and bell peppers, or adding spinach to your pasta dishes. Try out novel recipes with superfoods as the main ingredients. This not only adds variety to your meals but also ensures you're getting a wide range of nutrients.

Quick Superfood Recipes

To get you started on your superfood journey, here are a few quick and delicious recipes that you can easily incorporate into your daily routine:

Superfood Smoothie Bowl

Ingredients:

- 1 banana

- 1/2 cup frozen blueberries

- 1/2 cup spinach

- 1/2 avocado

- 1 cup almond milk

- 1 tablespoon chia seeds

- 1 tablespoon almond butter

Instructions:

1. Blend the banana, blueberries, spinach, avocado, and almond milk until smooth.

2. Pour the blended mixture into a bowl and top with chia seeds and almond butter.

3. Enjoy a nutritious and filling breakfast!

Quinoa Salad with Kale and Avocado

Ingredients:

- 1 cup cooked quinoa

- 2 cups chopped kale

- 1 avocado, diced

- 1/2 cup cherry tomatoes, halved

- 1/4 cup crumbled feta cheese

- 2 tablespoons olive oil

- 1 tablespoon lemon juice

- Salt and pepper to taste

Instructions:

1. In a large bowl, combine the quinoa, kale, avocado, cherry tomatoes, and feta cheese.

2. Trickle with olive oil and lemon juice, and season with salt and pepper.

3. Toss to combine and serve as a light and refreshing lunch or side dish.

Dark Chocolate and Almond Energy Bites

Ingredients:

- 1 cup rolled oats

- 1/2 cup almond butter

- 1/4 cup honey

- 1/4 cup dark chocolate chips

- 1/4 cup chopped almonds

- 1 tablespoon chia seeds

Instructions:

1. In a large bowl, combine the oats, almond butter, and honey until well combined.

2. Stir in the dark chocolate chips, chopped almonds, and chia seeds.

3. Fold the combination into little balls and refrigerate for no less than 30 minutes prior to serving.

4. Enjoy these as a healthy and satisfying snack!

By understanding the benefits of superfoods and incorporating them into your daily diet with these simple tips and recipes, you'll be well on your way to enhancing your health and well-being. Superfoods are an easy and delicious way to ensure you're getting the essential nutrients your body needs to thrive. So, let's embrace these nutritional powerhouses and enjoy the journey to better health, one delicious bite at a time

CHAPTER TWO

Nutritious Snacks on the Go

Importance of Healthy Snacking

In our fast-paced lives, it's easy to reach for convenient but unhealthy snacks. However, healthy snacking is crucial for maintaining energy levels, supporting metabolism, and preventing overeating during meals. Nutritious snacks can keep your blood sugar stable, improve mood, and enhance cognitive function, making them an essential part of a balanced diet.

Healthy snacking helps bridge the gap between meals and ensures your body receives a steady supply of nutrients throughout the day. Instead of relying on processed foods laden with sugar and unhealthy fats, choosing wholesome snacks can significantly impact your overall health and well-being.

Quick Snack Hacks

Finding time to prepare healthy snacks might seem challenging, but with a few quick hacks, you can make nutritious choices even on the busiest days.

1. **Prep in Advance**: Spend a few minutes each week preparing snack bags with nuts, seeds, or sliced fruits and vegetables. This makes it easy to grab a healthy snack when you're in a hurry.

2. **Portable Protein**: Keep portable protein sources like Greek yogurt, hard-boiled eggs, or small packets of nut butter on hand. Protein helps keep you full longer and supports muscle health.

3. **Healthy Trail Mix**: Create your own trail mix with a combination of nuts, seeds, dried fruits, and a few dark chocolate chips. This mix is a great source of healthy fats, fiber, and antioxidants.

4. **Fruit and Veggie Packs**: Slice fruits and vegetables like apples, carrots, celery, and bell peppers, and store them in the fridge for easy access. Pair them with hummus or a yogurt dip for added flavor and nutrition.

5. **Smoothie Packs**: Pre-pack smoothie ingredients in individual freezer bags. When you're ready for a snack, simply blend with your choice of liquid for a quick and nutritious smoothie.

Recipes for Nutritious Snacks

To help you incorporate healthy snacks into your routine, here are a few easy and delicious recipes:

Almond and Berry Yogurt Parfait

Ingredients:

- 1 cup Greek yogurt

- 1/2 cup each of strawberries, blueberries, raspberries, and strawberries)

- 1/4 cup granola

- 2 tablespoons sliced almonds

- 1 teaspoon honey (optional)

Instructions:

1. In a bowl or jar, layer half of the Greek yogurt, followed by half of the berries.

2. Add a layer of granola and sliced almonds.

3. Repeat the layers with the remaining yogurt and berries.

4. Drizzle with honey if desired. Enjoy this parfait as a refreshing and protein-packed snack.

Veggie Sticks with Hummus

Ingredients:

- 1 cup baby carrots

- 1 cup cucumber sticks

- 1 cup bell pepper strips

- 1/2 cup hummus

Instructions:

1. Arrange the baby carrots, cucumber sticks, and bell pepper strips on a plate or in a snack container.

2. Serve with hummus for dipping. This crunchy and satisfying snack is full of fiber and healthy fats.

Energy-Boosting Smoothie

Ingredients:

- 1 banana

- 1/2 cup frozen mango chunks

- 1/2 cup spinach

- 1/2 cup coconut water

- 1 tablespoon chia seeds

Instructions:

1. Put together all ingredients in a blender and blend until smooth.

2. Pour into a glass and enjoy this refreshing and energizing smoothie that's perfect for a midday boost.

Nut Butter Apple Sandwiches

Ingredients:

- 1 apple, cored and cut round

- 2 tablespoons almond or peanut butter

- 1 tablespoon raisins or dried cranberries

- 1 tablespoon granola

Instructions:

1. Spread a layer of nut butter on half of the apple slices.

2. Sprinkle with raisins or dried cranberries and granola.

3. Top with the remaining apple slices to make sandwiches. These apple sandwiches are a sweet and crunchy snack that's also filling and nutritious.

Overnight Oats with Berries

Ingredients:

- 1/2 cup rolled oats

- 1/2 cup almond milk

- 1/4 cup Greek yogurt

- 1/2 cup mixed berries

- 1 tablespoon chia seeds

- 1 teaspoon honey (optional)

Instructions:

1. In a jar or container, combine the rolled oats, almond milk, Greek yogurt, and chia seeds.

2. Stir well and top with mixed berries.

3. Drizzle with honey if desired.

4. Cover and refrigerate overnight. Enjoy this easy and portable snack the next day.

By understanding the importance of healthy snacking and incorporating these quick snack hacks and nutritious recipes into your daily routine, you can maintain your energy levels and support your overall health. These simple and delicious snacks are perfect for when you're on the go, ensuring you never have to compromise on nutrition, no matter how busy life gets.

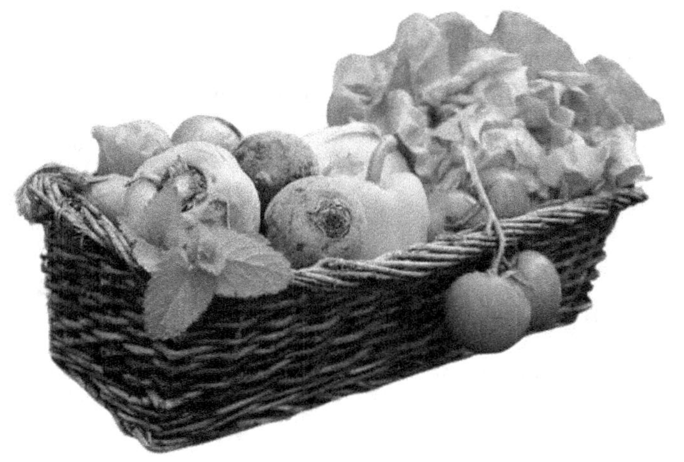

CHAPTER THREE

Delicious and Healthy Drinks

Hydration and Health

Maintaining adequate hydration is crucial to overall health and well-being. Water is the primary component of the human body and plays a crucial role in various bodily functions, including temperature regulation, digestion, and nutrient transport. Inadequate hydration can lead to fatigue, headaches, and impaired cognitive function. This chapter explores the importance of staying hydrated and introduces delicious drinks that can boost hydration while offering additional health benefits.

Easy Homemade Drinks

Creating homemade beverages is a fantastic way to ensure you're getting quality ingredients without added sugars or artificial additives. From refreshing infused waters to soothing herbal teas, homemade drinks can cater to your taste preferences and nutritional needs. Experiment with different combinations of fruits, herbs, and spices to discover your favorite flavors and enhance your hydration experience.

Citrus Infused Water

Ingredients:

- 1 lemon, thinly sliced

- 1 lime, thinly sliced

- 1 orange, thinly sliced

- Fresh mint leaves

- Ice cubes

- Water

Instructions:

1. Fill a pitcher with water.

2. Add the sliced lemon, lime, and orange.

3. Stir in a handful of fresh mint leaves.

4. Refrigerate for at least 1 hour to allow flavors to infuse.

5. Serve over ice. Enjoy this refreshing drink that is rich in vitamin C and antioxidants.

Herbal Iced Tea

Ingredients:

- 4 cups water

- 4 tea bags (e.g., chamomile, peppermint, or herbal blend)

- Honey or agave syrup (optional)

- Lemon slices (optional)

- Ice cubes

Instructions:

1. Boil water in a saucepan.

2. Remove from heat and add tea bags. Let steep for 5-10 minutes.

3. Remove tea bags and let the tea cool to room temperature.

4. Add honey or agave syrup if desired.

5. Refrigerate until chilled.

6. Serve over ice with lemon slices for a refreshing and soothing herbal tea.

Cucumber Mint Infused Water

Ingredients:

- 1 cucumber, thinly sliced

- Fresh mint leaves

- Ice cubes

- Water

Instructions:

1. Fill a pitcher with water.

2. Add the sliced cucumber and fresh mint leaves.

3. Refrigerate for at least 1 hour to infuse flavors.

4. Serve over ice. This hydrating drink is refreshing and helps to detoxify the body.

Ginger Lemonade

Ingredients:

- 4 cups water

- Juice of 4 lemons

- 1/2 cup honey or maple syrup

- 1 tablespoon freshly grated ginger

- Ice cubes

Instructions:

1. In a large pitcher, combine water, lemon juice, honey or maple syrup, and grated ginger.

2. Stir until honey or syrup is dissolved.

3. Refrigerate until chilled.

4. Serve over ice. This tangy and soothing drink is rich in vitamin C and aids digestion.

Berry Blast Smoothie

Ingredients:

- 1 cup of blended varieties of berries (strawberries, blueberries, raspberries)
- 1/2 banana
- 1/2 cup Greek yogurt
- 1/2 cup almond milk (or any choice of milk)
- 1 tablespoon chia seeds (optional)
- Ice cubes

Instructions:

1. Combine all ingredients in a blender.
2. Blend until smooth and creamy.
3. Pour into a glass and enjoy this antioxidant-packed smoothie that's perfect for a quick and nutritious snack.

Smoothies and Juices for Wellness

Smoothies and juices offer a convenient way to incorporate a variety of nutrients into your diet. Here are a couple of recipes for wellness:

Green Power Smoothie

Ingredients:

- 1 cup spinach leaves
- 1/2 cup kale leaves, stems removed
- 1/2 frozen banana
- 1/2 cup frozen mango chunks
- 1 tablespoon almond butter
- 1 cup coconut water (or your choice of liquid)

Instructions:

1. Add all ingredients to a blender.

2. Blend until smooth and creamy.

3. Pour into a glass and enjoy this nutrient-dense smoothie packed with vitamins, minerals, and fiber.

Refreshing Watermelon Mint Juice

Ingredients:

- 4 cups cubed seedless watermelon
- Juice of 1 lime
- Fresh mint leaves

- Ice cubes

Instructions:

1. In a blender, combine watermelon cubes and lime juice.

2. Blend until smooth.

3. Strain through a fine mesh sieve to remove pulp (optional).

4. Refrigerate until chilled.

5. Serve over ice with fresh mint leaves for a refreshing and hydrating drink.

Incorporate these delicious and healthy drink options into your daily routine to stay hydrated, support your wellness goals, and enjoy the benefits of nutritious beverages made at home. Whether you're looking for a refreshing drink to start your day or a satisfying smoothie post-workout, these recipes offer flavorful ways to enhance your hydration and overall health.

CHAPTER FOUR

Power Breakfasts with Cereals

With good reason, breakfast is regarded as the most important meal of the day. It sets the tone for your energy levels, metabolism, and overall well-being throughout the day. This chapter explores the significance of breakfast in maintaining a healthy lifestyle, focusing particularly on cereals as a nutritious choice.

The Role of Breakfast in Healthy Living

Breakfast jumpstarts your metabolism and provides the necessary energy to kickstart your day. It replenishes your glucose levels after a night of fasting, improving your concentration and mood. Research shows that individuals who regularly consume breakfast tend to have better overall nutrient intake and are more likely to maintain a healthy weight. By starting your day with a balanced breakfast, you set yourself up for success in achieving your health and wellness goals.

Choosing the Right Cereals

Selecting the right cereals is key to maximizing the benefits of your morning meal. Opt for whole grain cereals that offer a rich source of fibre, vitamins, and minerals. Avoid cereals with high sugar content and artificial additives, as these can lead to energy crashes and undermine your health goals. Reading nutrition labels empowers you to make informed choices, ensuring that your breakfast supports your dietary preferences and nutritional requirements.

Quick and Healthy Cereal Recipes

Embracing the convenience and versatility of cereals, quick and healthy recipes can transform your morning routine. From nourishing overnight oats to satisfying homemade granola and refreshing yogurt parfaits, these recipes are designed to fuel your body and tantalize your taste buds. By preparing wholesome breakfast options ahead of time, you set yourself up for success in maintaining a balanced diet and enjoying delicious meals that contribute to your overall well-being

Overnight Oats

Ingredients:

- 1/2 cup rolled oats

- 1/2 cup milk (dairy or plant-based)

- 1 tablespoon chia seeds

- 1/2 teaspoon vanilla extract

- 1 tablespoon honey or maple syrup (optional)

- Fresh berries or sliced bananas for topping

Instructions:

1. In a jar or bowl, combine rolled oats, milk, chia seeds, vanilla extract, and honey or maple syrup (if using).

2. Stir well to combine.

3. Cover and refrigerate overnight.

4. In the morning, stir the oats and add more milk if desired for desired consistency.

5. Top with fresh berries or sliced bananas before serving.

Homemade Granola

Ingredients:

- 2 cups rolled oats

- 1/2 cup nuts (almonds, walnuts, or pecans), chopped

- 1/4 cup seeds (pumpkin seeds or sunflower seeds)

- 1/4 cup honey or maple syrup

- 2 tablespoons coconut oil, melted

- 1/2 teaspoon vanilla extract

- 1/2 teaspoon ground cinnamon

- 1/4 teaspoon salt

- 1/2 cup dried fruits (cranberries, raisins, or chopped apricots)

Instructions:

1. Preheat oven to 300°F (150°C). Use material paper to line a baking sheet

2. In a large bowl, combine rolled oats, nuts, seeds, honey or maple syrup, melted coconut oil, vanilla extract, cinnamon, and salt. Mix until well combined.

3. Spread the mixture evenly onto the prepared baking sheet.

4. Bake for 25-30 minutes, stirring halfway through, until golden brown.

5. Remove from oven and allow it to cool completely.

6. Stir in dried fruits. Store in an airtight container.

Yogurt Parfait

Ingredients:

- 1 cup plain Greek yogurt

- 1/2 cup granola (store-bought or homemade)

- 1/2 cup fresh berries or sliced fruits (strawberries, blueberries, or bananas)

- Tickle honey or maple syrup (optional)

Instructions:

1. In a glass or bowl, layer Greek yogurt, granola, and fresh berries or sliced fruits.

2. Repeat the layers above until ingredients are used up.

3. Drizzle with honey or maple syrup if desired.

4. Serve immediately and enjoy this satisfying and nutritious breakfast parfait.

Incorporate these quick and healthy cereal recipes into your breakfast routine to start your day with a nutritious and satisfying meal. Whether you prefer overnight oats, homemade granola, or a refreshing yogurt parfait, these recipes provide delicious options to fuel your morning and support your health and well-being.

CHAPTER FIVE

Balanced and Tasty Meals

A healthy diet doesn't have to be hard or take a lot of time. This chapter explores the essentials of crafting meals that are not only nutritious but also delicious, offering practical tips and quick recipes to simplify your meal planning and preparation.

The Basics of a Balanced Meal

A balanced meal encompasses a combination of essential nutrients, including proteins, carbohydrates, healthy fats, vitamins, and minerals. This optimal blend supports overall health, regulates energy levels, and promotes satiety. To create a balanced plate, target including the following:

- **Proteins**: Lean meats, fish, poultry, tofu, beans, or legumes.
- **Carbohydrates**: Whole grains like quinoa, brown rice, and pasta made with whole wheat.

- **Healthy Fats**: Avocado, nuts, seeds, olive oil, or fatty fish like salmon.

- **Vegetables**: Colorful varieties rich in vitamins, minerals, and fiber.

- **Fruits**: Fresh or dried fruits for added antioxidants and natural sweetness.

By incorporating these elements into your meals, you provide your body with the nutrients it needs to thrive while enjoying a satisfying culinary experience.

Meal Prep Tips

Effective meal preparation is the cornerstone of maintaining a balanced diet amidst busy schedules. Consider these tips to streamline your meal prep process:

- **Plan Ahead**: Schedule dedicated time each week to plan meals and create a shopping list.

- **Batch Cooking**: Prepare larger quantities of staple ingredients like grains, proteins, and vegetables that can be used in multiple meals throughout the week.

- **Storage Solutions**: Invest in quality storage containers to keep prepped ingredients fresh and organized.

- **Variety and Flexibility**: Experiment with different flavors and ingredients to keep meals interesting and adaptable to changing tastes.

Quick and Easy Dinner Ideas

Transforming nutritious ingredients into flavorful meals doesn't have to be daunting. Try these quick and easy dinner ideas to inspire your culinary creativity:

- **One-Pot Pasta**: Combine whole-wheat pasta, vegetables, lean protein, and a homemade tomato sauce in a single pot for a hearty and nutritious meal.

- **Stir-Fry Delight**: Stir-fry lean protein, colorful vegetables, and whole grains like quinoa or brown rice with a dash of soy sauce or teriyaki for a savory, Asian-inspired dish.

- **Sheet Pan Suppers**: Roast a variety of vegetables with a lean protein (such as chicken or fish) on a sheet pan for an effortless yet satisfying meal.

By embracing balanced meal planning and preparation, you not only nourish your body with essential nutrients but also cultivate a sustainable approach to healthy eating. These practical strategies and delicious meal ideas empower you to enjoy flavorful dishes while supporting your overall well-being.

CHAPTER SIX

Sweet Treats without the Guilt

Indulging in sweet treats doesn't have to derail your healthy eating goals. This chapter explores ways to satisfy your sweet tooth with delicious desserts that are nutritious and guilt-free. Discover healthier dessert options, quick hacks for creating satisfying treats, and a collection of recipes that bring joy without compromising on your well-being.

Healthier Dessert Options

Choosing healthier dessert options is about making mindful choices that prioritize nutrition without sacrificing flavor. Consider these alternatives:

- **Fruit-Based Desserts**: Enjoy fresh fruit salads, fruit parfaits with yogurt, or baked apples with cinnamon for natural sweetness and vitamins.

- **Dark Chocolate**: Opt for dark chocolate with higher cocoa content, which is rich in antioxidants and lower in sugar compared to milk chocolate.

- **Frozen Yogurt**: Swap traditional ice cream for frozen yogurt made with Greek yogurt and fresh fruit toppings for a creamy, tangy treat.

Quick Dessert Hacks

When time is of the essence, these quick dessert hacks allow you to whip up a sweet treat in minutes:

- **Berry Bliss**: Combine mixed berries with a dollop of whipped coconut cream or Greek yogurt for a refreshing and satisfying dessert.

- **Nutty Delight**: Spread almond or peanut butter on apple slices and sprinkle with dark chocolate chips for a crunchy, nutrient-packed snack.

- **Banana "Ice Cream"**: Blend frozen bananas with a splash of almond milk and vanilla extract until smooth for a creamy, dairy-free alternative to ice cream.

Guilt-Free Sweet Recipes

Enjoy these guilt-free sweet recipes that bring joy to every bite while supporting your health goals:

- **Avocado Chocolate Mousse**: Blend ripe avocados with cocoa powder, honey or maple syrup, and a splash of almond milk until creamy. Chill and serve for a decadent yet nutritious dessert.

- **Chia Seed Pudding**: Almond milk, honey, vanilla extract, and chia seeds should be combined. For an extra crunch, top with fresh berries or nuts after letting it sit overnight to thicken.

- **Baked Cinnamon Apples**: Core apples and sprinkle with cinnamon and a drizzle of honey. For a warm and comforting dessert, bake until tender.

These recipes demonstrate that enjoying sweet treats can be part of a balanced diet. By incorporating healthier dessert options and quick hacks into your routine, you can satisfy cravings while maintaining a nutritious approach to eating. Embrace these guilt-free indulgences as part of your journey towards a healthier, happier lifestyle.

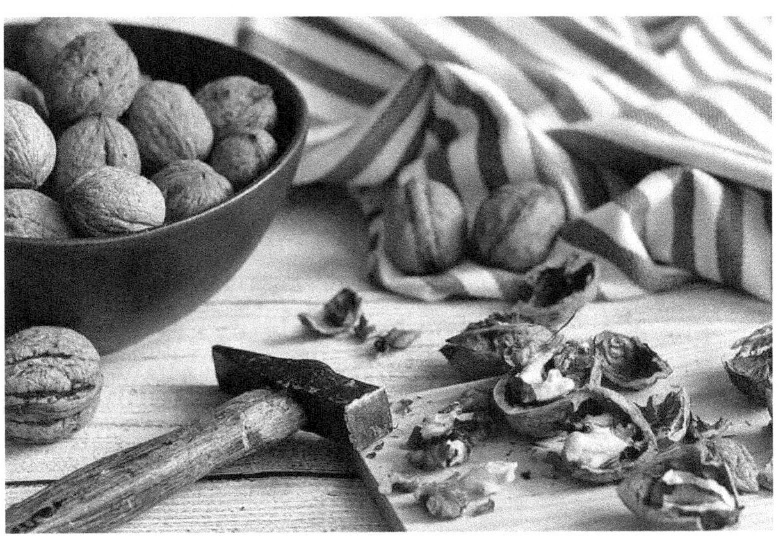

CHAPTER SEVEN

Savvy Grocery Shopping

Navigating the grocery store aisles with confidence is essential for maintaining a healthy and balanced diet. This chapter equips you with savvy tips and strategies for making informed choices, understanding nutrition labels, and selecting budget-friendly yet nutritious foods that support your wellness goals.

Shopping Tips for Healthy Eating

Transform your grocery shopping experience with these practical tips that prioritize health:

- **Plan Ahead**: Create a shopping list based on planned meals and snacks to avoid impulse purchases of unhealthy foods.
- **Shop the Perimeter**: Focus on fresh produce, lean meats, dairy, and whole grains typically found along the perimeter of the grocery store.

- **Read Ingredients**: Choose products with fewer ingredients, avoiding those with added sugars, trans fats, and artificial additives.

- **Buy in Bulk**: Purchase staple items like grains, beans, and frozen fruits/vegetables in bulk to save money and minimize shopping trips.

- **Shop Seasonally**: Opt for seasonal fruits and vegetables, which are often fresher, more flavorful, and less expensive.

Reading Nutrition Labels

Understanding nutrition labels empowers you to make informed decisions about the foods you buy:

- **Serving Size**: Pay attention to portion sizes as they dictate the nutritional content listed on the label.

- **Calories and Nutrients**: Monitor calories, fats (saturated and trans), sugars, sodium, and fiber to maintain a balanced diet.

- **Ingredients List**: Scan the ingredients list to identify potential allergens or additives and prioritize whole, recognizable ingredients.

Budget-Friendly Healthy Foods

Eating healthily doesn't have to break the bank. Explore these budget-friendly options for nutritious eating:

- **Whole Grains**: Choose affordable options like brown rice, oats, quinoa, and whole-wheat pasta for fiber and sustained energy.
- **Legumes**: Stock up on beans, lentils, and chickpeas, which are rich in protein, fiber, and essential nutrients.
- **Frozen Fruits and Vegetables**: Purchase frozen varieties for convenience without compromising nutritional value. They have a longer shelf life and are frequently more affordable.
- **Seasonal Produce**: Take advantage of seasonal fruits and vegetables, which are typically cheaper and more abundant.

By applying these savvy grocery shopping strategies, you can maximize your shopping efficiency, make healthier choices, and stay within your budget. Empower yourself with knowledge and smart shopping habits to support a balanced and nutritious diet that promotes overall well-being.

CHAPTER EIGHT

Kitchen Tips for Healthy Cooking

Efficient and healthy cooking begins with a well-equipped kitchen and smart techniques. This chapter explores essential tools, time-saving cooking methods, and tips for meal preparation and storage to streamline your culinary experience and support your healthy eating goals.

Essential Kitchen Tools for Quick Cooking

Equip your kitchen with these essential tools to simplify and expedite meal preparation:

- **Chef's Knife**: Invest in a high-quality chef's knife for chopping vegetables, fruits, and meats with ease and precision.
- **Cutting Board**: Use a durable cutting board that is large enough to comfortably chop ingredients and easy to clean.
- **Vegetable Peeler**: Opt for a sturdy vegetable peeler to quickly peel and prep vegetables for cooking.

- **Non-Stick Cookware**: Choose non-stick pans and pots to minimize the need for excess oils and fats during cooking.
- **Food Processor or Blender**: Utilize a food processor or blender for efficient chopping, pureeing, and blending of ingredients.

Time-Saving Cooking Techniques

Maximize efficiency in the kitchen with these time-saving techniques:

- **Batch Cooking**: Prepare large batches of grains, proteins, and vegetables at once to use throughout the week in various dishes.
- **One-Pot Meals**: Simplify cleanup and save time by cooking entire meals in a single pot or pan, such as soups, stews, and stir-fries.
- **Sheet Pan Dinners**: Roast a combination of vegetables and proteins on a sheet pan for a simple yet flavorful meal.

- **Slow Cooker or Instant Pot**: Use a slow cooker or Instant Pot for hands-off cooking that yields tender and delicious meals with minimal effort.

Meal Prep and Storage Tips

Efficient meal prep and storage practices ensure that healthy meals are readily available:

- **Prep Ingredients in Advance**: Wash, chop, and portion ingredients ahead of time to streamline meal preparation during busy weekdays.
- **Use Quality Storage Containers**: Invest in airtight containers for storing prepped ingredients and leftovers to maintain freshness.
- **Label and Organize**: Label containers with the contents and date to easily identify and rotate foods in your refrigerator or freezer.
- **Freeze Meals**: Prepare and freeze individual portions of meals for quick and convenient lunches or dinners.

By implementing these kitchen tips for healthy cooking, you can save time, minimize stress, and enjoy nutritious meals that support your overall well-being. Embrace efficient cooking techniques and organize your kitchen to make healthy eating a seamless part of your lifestyle.

CHAPTER NINE

Incorporating Fitness into Daily Life

Integrating regular physical activity into your daily routine is key to maintaining overall health and well-being. This chapter explores practical strategies for incorporating fitness into your busy schedule, including quick workouts, combining exercise with daily activities, and staying motivated to stay active.

Quick Workouts You Can Do Anywhere

Fit short bursts of exercise into your day with these convenient and effective workouts:

- **Bodyweight Exercises**: Perform exercises like squats, lunges, push-ups, and planks that require no equipment and can be done in small spaces.

- **High-Intensity Interval Training (HIIT)**: Alternate between periods of intense exercise (e.g., jumping jacks, burpees) and rest for a quick and efficient workout.

- **Walking or Jogging**: Take brisk walks or short jogs during breaks at work or in your neighborhood to boost cardiovascular health.

- **Stair Climbing**: Utilize stairs for a cardio workout that also strengthens leg muscles.

Combining Exercise with Daily Activities

Multitask by incorporating physical activity into your everyday routines:

- **Active Commuting**: Walk or bike to work, or park farther away from your destination to increase daily steps.

- **Household Chores**: Turn chores like vacuuming, gardening, or cleaning into opportunities to burn calories and stay active.

- **Desk Exercises**: Incorporate stretches and exercises at your desk to improve posture and circulation throughout the day.

Staying Motivated to Stay Active

Maintain enthusiasm for exercise with these motivational strategies:

- **Set Realistic Goals:** To stay motivated, set realistic fitness goals and track your progress.

- **Choose Activities You Enjoy:** Choose activities you enjoy, such as swimming, dancing, hiking, or playing a sport.

- **Accountability Partners**: Partner with a friend, family member, or fitness group to stay accountable and motivated.

- **Reward Yourself**: Celebrate milestones with non-food rewards, such as a new workout outfit or a relaxing massage.

By incorporating these strategies into your daily life, you can make fitness a natural and enjoyable part of your routine. Stay active, improve your health, and enhance your overall well-being with simple yet effective approaches to physical activity.

3.5

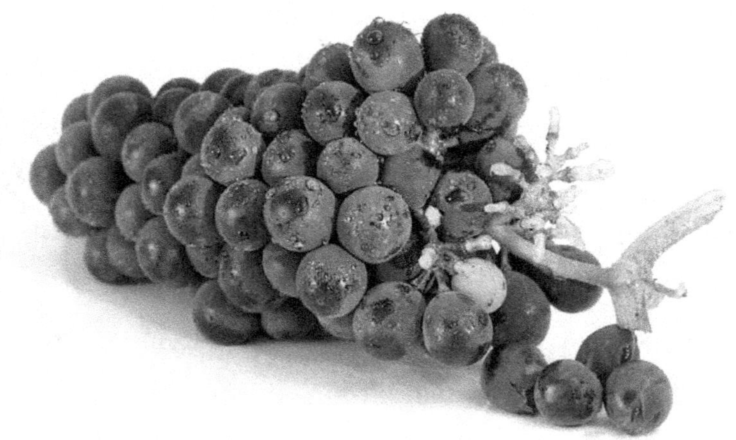

CHAPTER TEN

Mindful Eating and Living

In today's fast-paced world, practicing mindfulness in eating and daily life offers a transformative approach to health and well-being. This chapter explores the profound benefits of mindfulness, introduces mindful eating practices, and suggests practical ways to incorporate mindfulness into your routine for a balanced and fulfilling lifestyle.

The Benefits of Mindfulness

Mindfulness is more than a practice; it's a way of life that brings numerous benefits:

- **Stress Reduction**: Mindfulness helps alleviate stress by focusing on the present moment and cultivating a sense of calm.
- **Improved Eating Habits**: By becoming more aware of hunger and fullness cues, mindfulness promotes healthier eating habits and prevents overeating.

- **Enhanced Mental Clarity**: Regular mindfulness practice sharpens focus, enhances decision-making skills, and boosts cognitive function.

- **Emotional Regulation**: It fosters emotional resilience and helps manage difficult emotions effectively.

Mindful Eating Practices

Mindful eating involves paying full attention to the sensory experience of eating without judgment. Here are key mindful eating practices to cultivate:

- **Savoring**: Fully appreciate the flavors, textures, and aromas of your food with each bite.

- **Eating Slowly**: Take time to chew thoroughly and enjoy your meal, allowing your body to register fullness.

- **Listening to Hunger Cues**: Tune in to your body's signals of hunger and satiety to guide when and how much you eat.

- **Mindful Food Choices**: Make conscious decisions about what and how you eat, considering nutritional value and personal preferences.

Incorporating Mindfulness into Your Routine

Integrating mindfulness into daily life enhances overall well-being. Here's how to incorporate mindfulness practices into your routine:

- **Morning Meditation**: Begin your day with a couple of moments of contemplation to establish an inspirational vibe for the day ahead.
- **Mindful Breathing**: Practice mindful breathing exercises throughout the day to stay grounded and reduce stress.
- **Mindful Movement**: Incorporate activities like yoga or tai chi that emphasize mindful movement and body awareness.
- **Gratitude Practice**: Reflect on moments of gratitude each day to cultivate a positive mindset and appreciation for life.

By embracing mindfulness in eating and daily activities, you can cultivate a deeper connection with yourself and the world around you, leading to greater satisfaction and well-being in all aspects of life.

CHAPTER ELEVEN

Managing Stress Effectively

What is stress?

Stress is a natural response that our bodies have evolved to help us deal with challenges and threats. However, in today's fast-paced and often demanding world, chronic stress has become a significant health concern. Understanding its impact on our overall well-being is crucial for maintaining a healthy lifestyle.

At its core, stress triggers the body's "fight or flight" response, releasing hormones like adrenaline and cortisol to prepare us for action. While this response is essential in short bursts, prolonged exposure to stress can have detrimental effects on both our physical and mental health.

Physiologically, chronic stress can weaken the immune system, making us more susceptible to illnesses ranging from the common cold to more serious conditions like cardiovascular disease. It can also disrupt sleep patterns, which are vital for the body's repair and recovery processes.

Moreover, stress often manifests in unhealthy coping mechanisms such as overeating or indulging in comfort foods, smoking, excessive drinking, or neglecting physical activity. These behaviors can further exacerbate health issues and lead to weight gain, high blood pressure, and other chronic diseases.

On a mental and emotional level, chronic stress can contribute to anxiety, depression, irritability, and difficulty concentrating. It can strain relationships, reduce productivity, and diminish overall quality of life.

In the context of healthy living, managing stress effectively is essential. This involves adopting strategies to reduce stress levels, such as regular physical activity, mindfulness practices like meditation or deep breathing exercises, maintaining a balanced diet, getting adequate sleep, and seeking social support. These proactive steps not only help mitigate the negative effects of stress but also promote resilience and overall well-being.

Ultimately, recognizing the impact of stress on our health underscores the importance of incorporating stress management techniques into our daily routines. By doing so, we empower ourselves to lead healthier, more balanced lives and enhance our capacity to cope with life's challenges effectively.

Stress-Reducing Techniques

Not only is stress management important for our mental health but also for our overall health. Here's how incorporating stress-reducing techniques into your daily routine can pave the way to a healthier and happier life.

Firstly, practicing mindfulness and meditation can work wonders in calming the mind and reducing stress levels. Taking just a few minutes each day to breathe deeply, focus on the present moment, and clear your thoughts can significantly alleviate tension and promote relaxation.

Another effective method for reducing stress is physical activity. Engaging in regular exercise releases endorphins, the body's natural mood lifters, which help to reduce stress hormones like cortisol. Whether it's a brisk walk, yoga session, or a workout at the gym, finding an activity that you enjoy can serve as both a stress reliever and a boost to your overall fitness.

Furthermore, nurturing supportive relationships and social connections can provide invaluable emotional support during stressful times. Spending time with loved ones, sharing experiences, and seeking comfort in a strong support network can offer perspective and alleviate feelings of isolation.

Healthy eating habits also play a crucial role in managing stress. Consuming a balanced diet rich in fruits, vegetables, whole grains, and lean proteins provides your body with essential nutrients that support stress resilience. Avoiding excessive caffeine, sugar, and processed foods can help stabilize mood and energy levels throughout the day.

Lastly, incorporating relaxation techniques such as deep breathing exercises, progressive muscle relaxation, or indulging in hobbies and activities that bring you joy can further enhance your ability to cope with stress.

By integrating these stress-reducing techniques into your daily routine, you're not only taking proactive steps towards managing stress but also promoting a healthier lifestyle overall. Remember, prioritizing your mental and emotional well-being is an investment in yourself and your future happiness.

CHAPTER TWELVE

Creating Your Healthy Living Plan

Now that you've gathered insights and strategies for a healthier lifestyle, it's time to craft your personalized Healthy Living Plan. This plan will serve as your roadmap to achieving your health goals and maintaining a balanced and fulfilling life. You can create your plan by doing the following:

1. Define Your Goals

- **Health Objectives**: Identify specific health goals such as weight management, increased energy levels, or improved fitness.
- **Timeline**: Set realistic timelines for achieving each goal to keep yourself accountable and motivated.
- **Priorities**: Determine which aspects of health are most important to you and prioritize them in your plan.

2. Assess Your Current Lifestyle

- **Health Assessment**: Evaluate your current eating habits, physical activity level, stress management practices, and sleep patterns.
- **Identify Challenges**: Recognize any obstacles or habits that may hinder your progress towards a healthier lifestyle.

3. Nutrition and Diet

- **Balanced Meals**: Plan meals that include a variety of nutrient-dense foods such as fruits, vegetables, whole grains, lean proteins, and healthy fats.
- **Portion Control**: Practice mindful eating and portion control to maintain a healthy weight and support digestion.
- **Meal Preparation**: Schedule time for meal preparation to ensure you have nutritious meals ready when you need them.

4. Physical Activity

- **Exercise Routine**: Choose physical activities you enjoy and can sustain, aiming for at least 150 minutes of moderate-intensity aerobic activity per week.
- **Incorporate Movement**: Find opportunities to incorporate physical activity into your daily routine, such as walking or cycling to work, taking the stairs, or doing home workouts.

5. Stress Management

- **Stress Reduction Techniques**: Incorporate stress-reducing practices such as mindfulness meditation, deep breathing exercises, yoga, or spending time in nature.
- **Time for Relaxation**: Schedule regular breaks and downtime to recharge and prevent burnout.

6. Sleep Quality

- **Sleep Hygiene**: Establish a bedtime routine and create a sleep-friendly environment to improve the quality and duration of your sleep.

- **Consistent Sleep Schedule**: Aim for seven to nine hours of sleep per night to support overall health and well-being.

7. Hydration

- **Water Intake**: Drink an adequate amount of water throughout the day to stay hydrated and support bodily functions.
- **Avoid Sugary Drinks:** Avoid sugary drinks and instead drink water, herbal teas, or infused water.

8. Monitoring and Accountability

- **Track Progress**: Keep a journal or use apps to track your food intake, physical activity, and mood.
- **Regular Check-ins**: Schedule regular check-ins with yourself to assess your progress, adjust goals as needed, and celebrate your achievements.

9. Seek Support

- **Community and Resources**: Join support groups, fitness classes, or online communities to connect with others who share similar health goals.
- **Professional Guidance**: Consult with healthcare professionals, such as dietitians or personal trainers, for personalized advice and support.

10. Stay Motivated

- **Visualize Success**: Visualize yourself achieving your health goals and remind yourself of the benefits of a healthy lifestyle.
- **Reward Yourself**: Celebrate milestones along the way with non-food rewards that reinforce positive behaviors.

By creating and following your Healthy Living Plan, you empower yourself to make lasting changes that promote overall health, vitality, and well-being. Embrace this journey towards a healthier you, one step at a time.

Encouragement and Final Thoughts

Remember, embarking on a journey towards better health requires dedication and perseverance. Below are some words of encouragement:

- **You Can Do It**: Believe in yourself and your ability to make positive changes.
- **Celebrate Every Step**: Celebrate your successes, big or small, and acknowledge your efforts.
- **Stay Inspired**: Surround yourself with supportive friends, family, or communities who share your commitment to health.
- **Embrace Balance**: Find balance in your life by nurturing both your physical and mental well-being.

As you move forward, know that each step you take towards a healthier lifestyle is a step towards a happier, more fulfilling life. Stay committed, stay motivated, and enjoy the journey to vibrant health and well-being.

CONCLUSION

In conclusion, "Healthy Living Hacks: Quick Tips for a Better Life" serves as your comprehensive guide to transforming everyday habits into pathways to wellness. Throughout this journey, we've explored practical strategies to enhance your health, from nutritious meal ideas and mindful eating practices to quick workout routines and stress-reducing techniques.

The essence of this book lies in its simplicity and effectiveness. By incorporating these hacks into your daily routine, you're not just improving your physical health but also nurturing your mental and emotional well-being. Each tip is designed to be easy to implement, ensuring that health-conscious choices become second nature.

Remember, the key to sustainable health is consistency and self-awareness. Listen to your body, celebrate your progress, and embrace the journey towards a healthier lifestyle with enthusiasm. Whether you're striving to manage weight, boost energy levels, or simply adopt healthier habits, every small change contributes to your overall well-being.

As you continue on your path, keep experimenting with new recipes, staying active, and prioritizing self-care. Let this book be your companion in achieving balance and vitality in all aspects of life. Your health is your greatest asset, and by making informed choices today, you're investing in a brighter, healthier tomorrow.

Thank you for joining me on this journey towards better health. May these healthy living hacks empower you to live your best life, full of vitality, happiness, and wellness. Here's to a future filled with energy, resilience, and the joy of living well!